Narjes ABID

Impact of smoking on lung disease COVID-19

Narjes ABID

Impact of smoking on lung disease COVID-19

ScienciaScripts

Imprint

Cover image: www.ingimage.com

This book is a translation from the original published under ISBN 978-620-6-72330-1.

Publisher:
Sciencia Scripts
is a trademark of
Dodo Books Indian Ocean Ltd. and OmniScriptum S.R.L publishing group

120 High Road, East Finchley, London, N2 9ED, United Kingdom
Str. Armeneasca 28/1, office 1, Chisinau MD-2012, Republic of Moldova, Europe
Printed at: see last page
ISBN: 978-620-8-34015-5

Thanks

To my dear friend and President of the Jury Professor Gargouri Imen

Thank you for having honored me by agreeing to chair this jury.

Please find in this work the testimony of my friendship and my most sincere thanks.

To Madame and Judge DR OMRANE Asma

Thank you for agreeing to sit on the Jury for this dissertation.

Please find in this work the expression of my deepest thanks

To my dear friend and thesis supervisor Associate Professor Loukil Manel

Thank you, dear friend, for your invaluable advice and availability.

Please find in this work the testimony of my friendship and my most sincere thanks.

TABLE OF CONTENTS

LIST OF ABBREVIATIONS

SARS-CoV-2 : Severe Acute Respiratory Syndrome-Coronavirus 2

COVID-19: Coronavirus Disease 2019 (COronaVIrus Disease 2019)

RT-PCR : Reverse Transcription - Polymerase Chain Reaction

PA pack-years

BMI : body mass index

SpO2 pulsed oxygen saturation

SPSS Statistical Package for Social Science

G1 Group 1

G2 : Group 2

WHO : World Health Organization

ACE2: angiotensin converting enzyme 2

INTRODUCTION

INTRODUCTION

Severe Acute Respiratory Syndrome-Coronavirus 2 or SARS-CoV-2 causing Coronavirus Disease 2019 (COronaVIrus Disease 2019 or COVID-19) was responsible for the biggest infectious pandemic since the Spanish flu of 1918. The disease primarily affects the respiratory system, with polymorphous clinical pictures ranging from asymptomatic forms to acute respiratory distress syndrome (1). Several studies have been carried out to determine the prognostic factors for morbidity and mortality in this condition. Some of these factors may be useful in guiding therapeutic management.(2). It is well established that smoking is responsible for significant cardiovascular and respiratory morbidity. It is one of the world's leading causes of avoidable mortality. However, the clinical, radiological and evolutionary impact of smoking on SARS-CoV-2 pneumonia remains controversial. (3).

The main aim of our work was to assess the impact of smoking on the radio-clinical presentation of COVID-19 pneumopathy, and to determine its influence on the evolution of this condition.

METHODS

METHODS

1. TYPE AND DURATION OF STUDY

This is a retrospective descriptive study involving patients who were hospitalized for COVID-19 pneumopathy at the Pneumology Department at Mohamed Taher Maamouri Hospital Nabeul during the period from September 2020 to March 2021.

2. INCLUSION CRITERIA

- Age 18 and over
- SARS-CoV-2 infection confirmed by rapid antigen test or Transcription reverse polymerase chain reaction (RT-PCR) and having a respiratory impact defined by the presence of clinical and/or radiological signs secondary to this infection.

3. NON-INCLUSION CRITERIA

- COVID-19 infection based on clinical and/or radiological presumption and not virologically confirmed
- Confirmed COVID-19 infection without respiratory involvement
- Patient's smoking status not specified

4. EXCLUSION CRITERIA

- Concurrent parenchymal respiratory pathology

5. DATA COLLECTION

- A worksheet was drawn up to collect data from each patient (Appendix 1).
- The data collected included:

5.1. Characteristics of patients

The following were collected:

- Socio-demographic data: age, gender
- Smoking pack-years (PA)
- The anthropometric parameters: weight, height and body mass index (BMI). Obesity is defined as a BMI greater than or equal to 30kg/m^2, Overweight is defined as a BMI between 25 and 30 kg/m^2
- Comorbidities
- Long-term treatment

5.2. Characteristics of COVID-19 pneumopathy

5.2.1. Clinical data

- Respiratory and extra-respiratory functional signs
- Clinical examination data: presence of signs of respiratory struggle (polypnea, supra-sternal and inter-costal tugging, thoracoabdominal rocking), initial level of pulsed oxygen saturation (SpO2)

5.2.2. Assessment of severity

- A severe form is defined by the presence of a room air SpO2 of less than 90% and/or signs of respiratory struggle. (4).

5.2.3. Radiological data

Data collected from chest scans performed during hospitalization for COVID-19 pneumonitis included:

- Type of lesions: ground glass, condensation
- Ground glass is defined as an increase in the density of the lung parenchyma. The vessels within it remain visible and of normal caliber. (5).

- Parenchymal condensation corresponds to an increase in lung density that obliterates vessel contours, unlike ground-glass hyperdensities.(5).
- Extent of scanographic lesions assessed using the visual quantification scale of the Société Française de Radiologie: minimal (< 10%), moderate (10-25%), extensive (25-50%), severe (50-75%), critical (> 75%). (6).

5.2.1. Therapeutic data

- Use of oxygen therapy and flow rate. For each patient we have noted the maximum flow rate required.)
- Prescription and duration of systemic corticosteroid therapy

5.2.2. Evolutionary data

The following data were collected

- Length of hospital stay
- The occurrence of respiratory or extra-respiratory complications
- A possible stay in intensive care
- Discharge from hospital with or without oxygen
- The number of patients who died

6. STATISTICAL ANALYSIS :

Data were entered and analyzed using SPSS (Statistical Package for Social Science) version 20 software.

6.1. DESCRIPTIVE STUDY

- Quantitative values are expressed as mean and standard deviation.
- Qualitative values were expressed in terms of frequency and number of employees.

6.2. ANALYTICAL STUDY

For the statistical analysis and comparative study, the following tests were used:

- The STUDENT test for independent quantitative values.
- The KHI2 test for qualitative values.

The difference is considered statistically significant when p is less than 0.05.

6.3. LITERATURE SEARCH

We used the search engine: pubmed.ncbi.nlm.nih.gov and the following bibliographic search site: www.sciencedirect.com

6.4. ETHICAL CONSIDERATIONS

We declare that we have no conflict of interest in this study and that medical confidentiality has been respected.

RESULTS

RESULTS

During the study period, 383 patients were hospitalized with COVID-19 pneumonia confirmed by RT-PCR. One hundred and sixteen patients whose smoking status was not specified were not included. Of the remaining 267 patients, 30 patients with respiratory pathology and parenchymal involvement were excluded.

A total of 237 patients were included in our study.

1. DESCRIPTIVE STUDY

1.1 PATIENT CHARACTERISTICS

1.1.1. Socio-demographic characteristics

1.1.1.1. Age

The mean age of our patients was 62.7 ±13.7 years with extremes ranging from 18 to 92 years.

1.1.1.2. Gender

Our population comprised 128 men (54%) and 109 women (46%) (Figure 1).

The sex ratio was 1.17

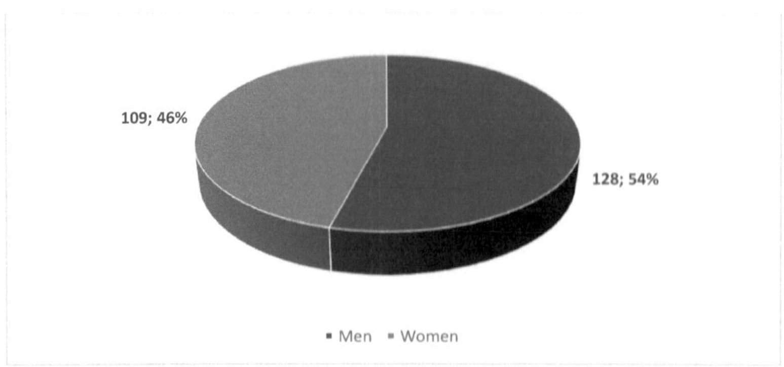

Figure 1: Breakdown of study population by gender

1.1.1.3. Tobacco

In our study, 53 patients (22.4%) were smokers.

The mean smoking intake in BP was 33±22 BP with extremes from 2 to 100 BP and a median of 30 BP.

Twenty-six patients were weaned at the time of the study.

1.1.2. Anthropometric parameters

The average weight of our population was 81.2 ± 16.2 kg [41-140].

The mean BMI was 29.5 ± 5.3 kg/m^2 with extremes ranging from 16.8 to 51 kg/m^2

Ninety-two patients were obese (38.8%) and 107 patients were overweight (45.1%) (Figure 2).

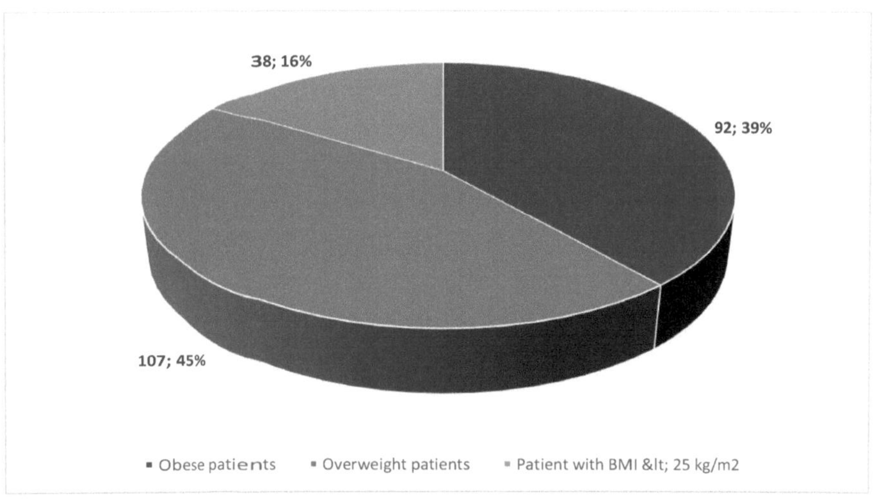

Figure 2: Distribution of the study population according to corpulence

1.1.3. Comorbidities

Almost three-quarters of patients had at least one comorbidity (164; 69.2%).

A history of diabetes was found in 93 cases (39.2%), insulin-requiring in

30 cases (12.6%)

Cardiovascular comorbidities were present in almost half of cases (56.1%). They included arterial hypertension in 121 cases (51.1%), coronary insufficiency in 19 cases (8%), arrhythmia in 10 cases (4.2%) and heart failure in 7 cases (3%).

Thirteen patients had chronic renal failure (5.5%) and one patient had cirrhosis.

A history of neoplasia was found in 7 cases: multiple myeloma (2 cases), lymphoma (1 case), breast carcinoma (1 case), colonic neoplasia (1 case), basal cell carcinoma (1 case) and prostatic adenocarcinoma (1 case).

Seven patients were treated for hypothyroidism and one for Wegener's disease.

1.1.4. Long-term treatment

Thirty patients were on insulin (12.6%)

Seven patients were on long-term corticosteroid therapy

Sixty patients had at least one antihypertensive treatment (ACE inhibitor 27 cases (11.4%); angiotensin II receptor antagonists 33 cases (13.9%)).

1.2 CHARACTERISTICS OF COVID PNEUMOPATHY

1.2.1. Clinical data

1.2.1.1. Clinical warning signs

1.2.1.1.1. Respiratory and extra-respiratory functional signs (Figure 2)

Respiratory signs were present in the majority of cases (203 cases; 85.6%). They were dominated by dyspnea, present in 176 cases (74.3%), followed by cough, reported in 151 cases (63.7%). Chest pain was present in 25 cases (10.5%).

Digestive signs included diarrhea in 27 cases (11.4%), abdominal pain in 17 cases (7.2%), and nausea and/or vomiting in 28 cases (11.8%).

Myalgias were present in 51 cases (21.5%) and arthralgias in 49 cases (20.7%).

Thirteen patients complained of agueusia (5.5%) and 17 patients (7.2%) of anosmia.

1.2.1.1.2. General signs

General signs were present in 80.16% of cases (190 patients), dominated by fever (136 cases; 57.4%), followed by asthenia in 121 cases (51.1%).

1.2.1.2. Physical examination data

Signs of respiratory struggle were present in 11 cases (4.6%).

SpO2 on admission to room air averaged 87±5.9%, with extremes ranging from 60 to 99%.

Just under half of patients (108 patients, 45.5%) had SpO2<90% with a mean saturation of 84% [60-89].

1.2.1.3. Severity classification

About half the cases were severe (109 cases, 46%).

1.2.2. Radiological data

Chest CT scans were performed on 155 patients (65.7%).

Parenchymal involvement related to COVID-19 pneumopathy was observed in 150 cases (96.7%).

The main CT abnormalities found were ground glass (126 cases; 81.29%) and condensations (85 cases; 54.8%) of peripheral and subpleural distribution. These two anomalies were associated in 74 cases (47.7%).

The extent of lesions was critical in 31 cases (20%), severe in 49 cases (31.6%) and absent in 6 cases (3.8%) (Figure 3).

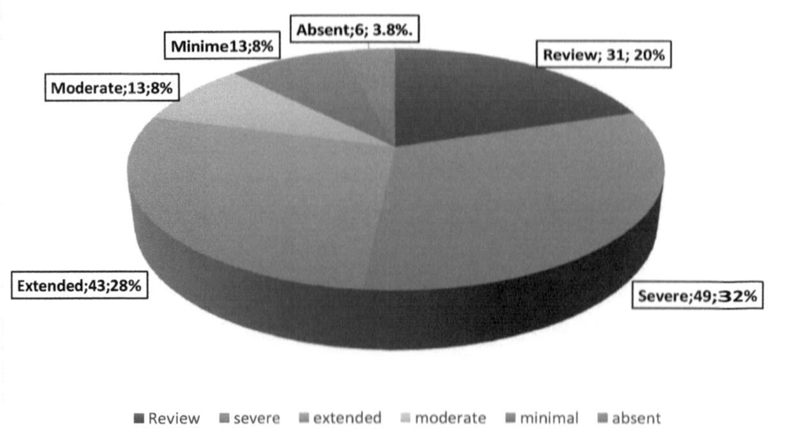

Figure 3: Distribution of study population according to extent of CT lesions

Pulmonary embolism was observed in 42 patients (42/155; 27%).

1.2.3. Therapeutic data

Oxygen therapy was required for 204 patients (86%) with a mean flow rate of 10.8 l/min [2-60].

For 133 patients (56.1%), the oxygen flow rate was greater than or equal to 6l/min.

Dexamethasone-based systemic corticosteroid therapy was prescribed for 217 patients (92.8%).

The prescribed dose was 6 mg in almost half of cases (44.7%) (Figure 4).

The average duration of corticosteroid therapy was 10.76±6.5 days.

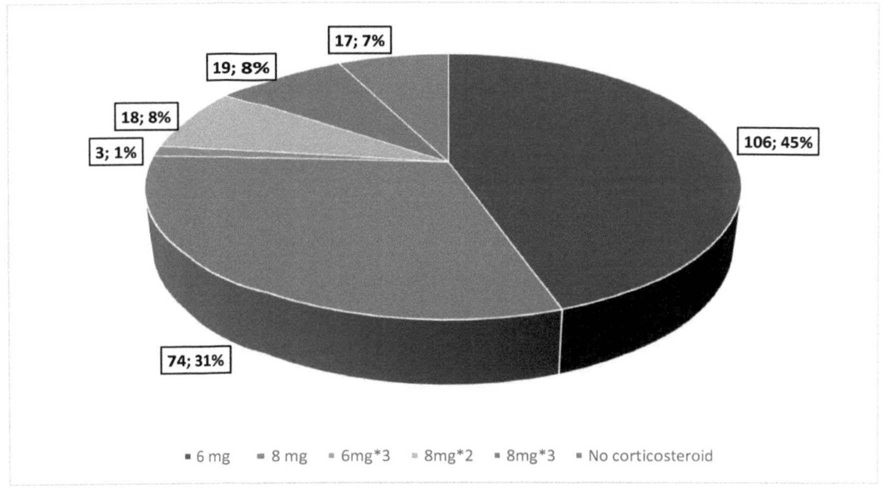

Figure 4: Distribution of study population by dose of corticosteroid therapy prescribed (Dexamethasone)

1.2.4. Evolutionary data

1.2.4.1. Occurrence of complications

Pulmonary embolism was diagnosed in 42 cases (17.7%). It was unilateral in two cases and bilateral in 40. Its location was distal in 38 patients and proximal in four others.

Bronchial superinfection was noted in 39 cases (16.4%).

Cardiac complications occurred in 25 cases (10.5%), including rhythm disorders (8 cases), acute coronary syndrome (8 cases), advanced heart failure (13 cases) and myocarditis (1 case).

1.2.4.2. Evolution

Seventy-four patients (31.2%) required a stay in intensive care.

Sixteen patients died (6.75%)

Mean room air SpO2 at discharge was 95.39±2.13% [84-99%]

Thirteen patients required oxygen therapy at discharge (5.4%)

2. ANALYTICAL STUDY

The study population was divided into two groups (Figure 5)

- Group 1 (G1) group of non-smoking patients: 184 patients (77.6%)
- Group 2 (G2) group of smoking patients: 53 patients (22.4%)

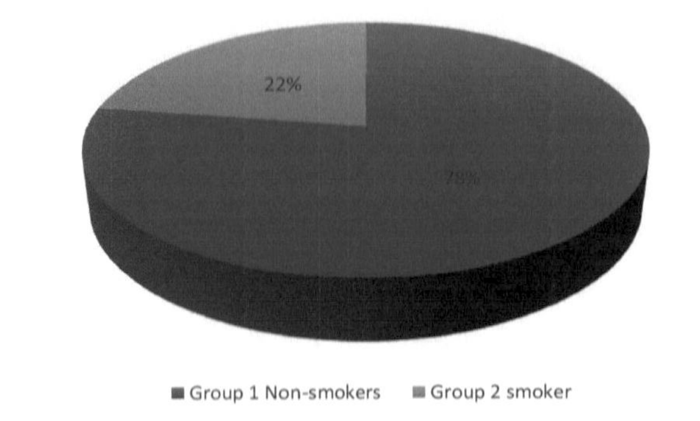

Figure 5: Breakdown of study population by smoking status

2.1. SOCIO-DEMOGRAPHIC CHARACTERISTICS

2.1.1. Age

The mean age for smoking patients was 61.1 ± 12.9 years [26-89 years], whereas it was 63.2±13.9 for non-smoking patients [18-92 years] ($p=0.322$).

2.1.2. Gender

The first group was predominantly female (108 women, 76 men; $p<0.001$), while the second group was predominantly male (52 men and one woman; $p<0.001$) (Figure 6).

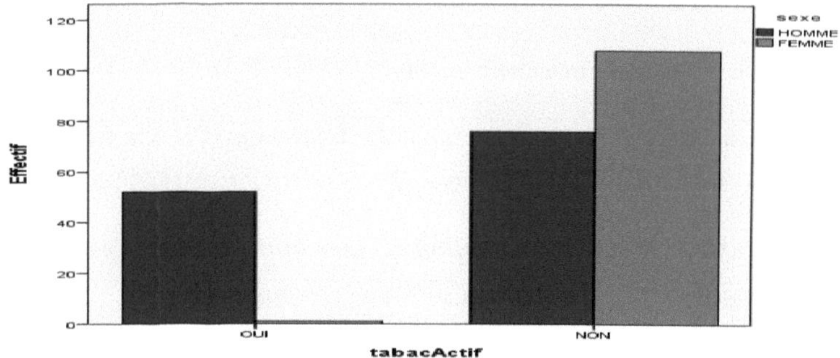

Figure 6: Gender distribution of the two groups studied

2.2 ANTHROPOMETRIC CHARACTERISTICS

There were more obese patients in the first group than in the second (79 (42%) versus 13 (24.5%); p=0.015).

The proportion of overweight patients was comparable for both groups (G1: 104 patients (56.6%) versus G2 26 patients (49%); p=0.336).

2.3 COMORBIDITIES

The distribution of the various comorbidities was comparable for both groups (Figure 7).

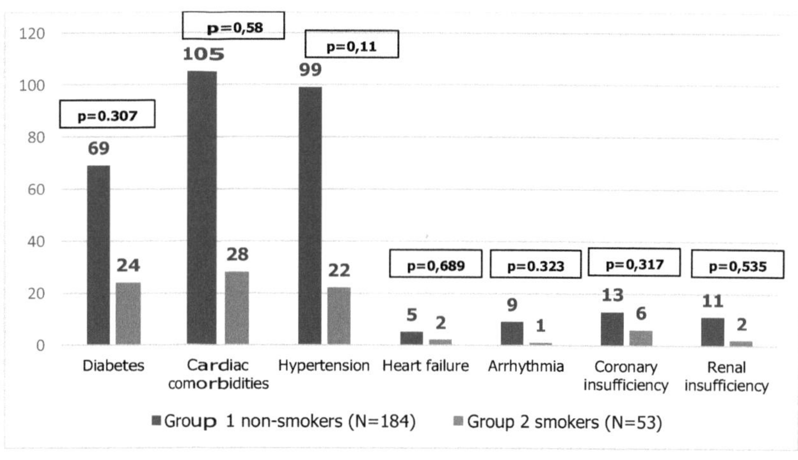

Figure 7: Distribution of comorbidities in the two study groups

2.4. CLINICAL DATA (TABLE I)

Fever and chest pain were more frequent in group 2.

There was no statistically significant difference in the frequency of severe forms between the two groups (G1 84 severe forms (45.6%) versus G2 25 severe forms (47.1%); p=0.845).

Table I: Distribution of clinical signs in the two groups

Clinical sign	*Group 1*	*Group 2*	*p*
Fever	99 (53,8%)	37 (69,8%)	**0,025**
Asthenia	92 (50%)	29 (54,7%)	0,462
Dry cough	121 (65,7%)	30 (56,6%)	0,285
Dyspnea	140 (76,1%)	36 (67,9%)	0,316
Chest pain	15 (8%)	10 (18,8%)	**0,022**
Nausea and/or vomiting	19 (10,3%)	9 (16,9%)	0,169
Abdominal pain	12 (6,5%)	5 (9,4%)	0,446
Diarrhea	21 (11,4%)	6 (11,3)	0,98
Agueusia	11 (5,9%)	2 (3,7%)	0,552
Anosmia	15 (8,1%)	2 (3,7%)	0,289
SpO2	87,6%	88,4%	0,442
Signs of respiratory struggle	10 (5,4%)	1(1,8%)	0,305

Group 1: non-smoking patients (n=184)

Group 2: group of smoking patients (n=53)

2.5. RADIOLOGICAL DATA

Chest CT scans were performed on 123 patients in the first group (66.8%) and 32 patients in the second group (60.3%) (p=0.476).

It showed abnormalities in favor of COVID-19 pneumopathy in 119/123 cases of G1 (96.7%) and 31/32 cases of G2 (96.8%) (p=0.971).

2.5.1. Type of radiological lesions

Ground glass and condensation were found to be comparable in both groups (Figure 8).

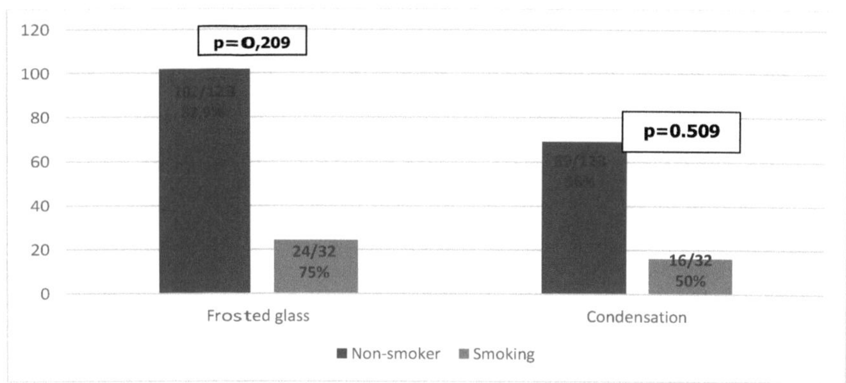

Figure 8: Distribution of CT lesions between the two groups studied

2.5.2 Extent of lesions

There was no statically significant difference in the distribution of lesion extent between the two groups studied (Figure 9).

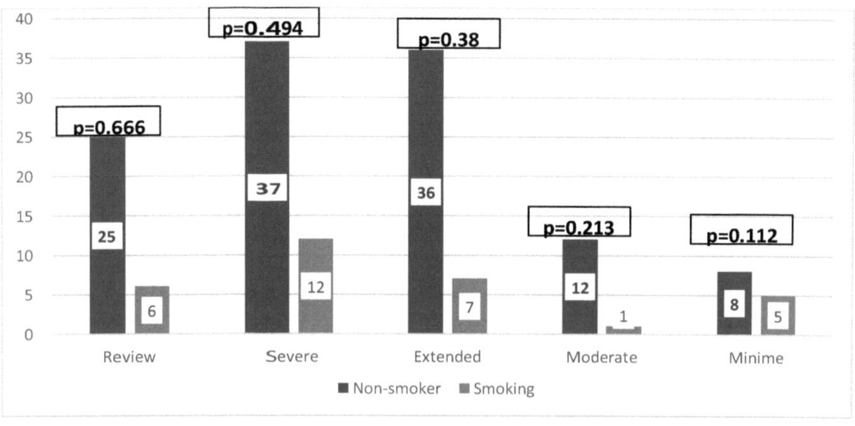

Figure 9: Distribution of the extent of radiological lesions according to the two groups studied

2.6. THERAPEUTIC DATA :

Oxygen therapy was required in both groups with no statistically significant difference (G1: 159 patients (86.4%) versus G2: 45 patients (84.9%); p=0.780).

Initial oxygen flow for the first group was 8.7±9.2 l/min and for the second group 11.2 ±13.2 l/min (p=0.124).

A flow rate greater than 6l/min was required for 96 patients in group 1 (52.1%) and 27 patients in group 2 (50%) (p=0.978).

There was no statistically significant difference in the prescription of corticosteroid therapy between the two groups studied (G1: 169 patients (91.8%) versus G2: 51 patients (96.2%); p=0.276), nor in its duration (G1 10.5±5.7 days versus G2 11.5 ±8.6 days; p=0.337).

2.7. EVOLUTIONARY DATA

Bronchial superinfection with recourse to antibiotic therapy was more frequent in the smoking group, with a statically significant difference (G1 24 cases (13%) versus G2 15 cases (28.3%); p=0.008).

The incidence of pulmonary embolism was similar in both groups (G1 37 cases (20.1%) versus G2 5 cases (9.4%); p=0.073). The same was true of cardiac complications (G1 21 cases (11.4%) versus G2 4 cases (7.5%); p=0.419).

There was no statically significant difference in mean room air SpO2 at discharge between the two groups (G1 95.4±2.14% versus G2 95.14±2.12%; p=0.391).

Death rates and ICU stays for both groups (Table II)

Table II: Comparison of evolutionary data by smoking status

Clinical sign	*Group 1*	*Group 2*	*p*
Deaths	14 (7,6%)	2 (3,7%)	0,327
Stay in intensive care	58 (31,5%)	16 (30,2%)	0,854

Discussion

DISCUSSION

The COVID-19 pandemic was declared by the World Health Organization (WHO) on March 11, 2020. Since then, it has been the source of heavy morbidity and mortality, with 774 million cases officially recorded, causing 7 million deaths by March 2024. (7). It then became a major public health problem, like tobacco, which is responsible for over 8 million deaths a year (8). Several studies have assessed the relationship between tobacco and COVID-19, with sometimes contradictory results.

The aim of our study was to assess the impact of smoking on the radio-clinical presentation of COVID-19 pneumopathy and to clarify its influence on its evolution.

Our study population comprised 237 patients, 184 of whom were smokers and 53 non-smokers. It was predominantly male, with a sex ratio of 1.17 and a mean age of 62.7 ±13.7 years. Apart from obesity, which was more frequent in smokers, the two groups were comparable in terms of comorbidity, namely diabetes, arterial hypertension, heart failure, arrhythmia and coronary insufficiency. The main clinical respiratory signs were dry cough and dyspnoea, which were equally present in both groups. The extent of CT lesions, consisting of ground glass sometimes associated with peripheral and subpleural condensation, was similar in both groups. Smokers and non-smokers had comparable rates of cardiac complications and pulmonary embolism, but smokers developed bronchial superinfections more often.

Rates of death and resuscitation were comparable between the two groups.

Highlights of our study

- The relatively large size of the study population
- This is a topical issue that is a major concern for global health.

Weaknesses of our study :

- Retrospective data collection
- Its monocentric nature

Several observational studies have shown a lower prevalence of smokers among subjects infected with SARS-CoV-2. Guan et al. in their study of 1099 patients admitted to a Chinese hospital with COVID-19 infection, found that ex-smokers and active smokers accounted for

1.9% and 12.6% of cases respectively (9). In another French study, the daily incidence of smokers among patients hospitalized for a COVID-19 infection was 4.4%, and that of patients with the same condition but not hospitalized was 5.3%. (10). A large, recently updated meta-analysis confirms this low prevalence. In this meta-analysis, active smokers had a lower risk of testing positive for SARS-CoV-2 than never smokers (11). The same finding was found in our study, with smokers representing only 22% of our population. This low prevalence has led researchers to conclude that smoking may have a "protective effect" against SARS-CoV-2 infection. (12). The main hypothesis put forward in the literature to explain this effect is based on the anti-inflammatory properties of nicotine . In fact, nicotine is an acetylcholine receptor agonist with an inhibitory action on cholinergic pro-inflammatory cytokines such as TNF, IL-1 and IL-6, without inhibiting the production of anti-inflammatory cytokines such as interleukin 10 (13,14). It would therefore prevent the cytokine storm and consequently the macrophagic activation syndrome caused by SARS-CoV-2 infection (15,16). The other explanation found was based on the fact that SARS-CoV-2 uses angiotensin-converting enzyme 2 (ACE2) as a receptor for entry into the cell (17) and that nicotine inhibits ACE2 expression, hence its protective effect against this virus (18,19). These findings led researchers to suggest a potential therapeutic effect of nicotine and nicotine substitutes against this viral infection (13,14).

These data have not been unanimously accepted, and have been the subject of much criticism. According to some authors, the low prevalence of smokers among subjects infected with SARS-CoV-2 is due to the quality of the data collected on smoking status, which is sometimes incomplete because it is often obtained retrospectively from medical records, which can be unreliable and biased because the data is often collected in a hurry. (3). Because of its retrospective nature, our study suffers from the same methodological bias. Indeed, during the period of our work, 116 patients hospitalized for COVID-19 pneumonia were not included due to lack of information on their smoking status.

The "protective effect" of nicotine has also been questioned by some authors, who argue that tobacco smoke has a deleterious effect on the respiratory epithelium. It reduces its immune defences and alters mucociliary clearance, thereby increasing the risk of viral and bacterial infections. What's more, recent research has shown that nicotine induces overexpression of ACE2, thus promoting the entry of SARS-CoV-2 into the body (20). Furthermore, tobacco plays a definite role in the development of comorbidities, especially cardiovascular ones, which are factors in the unfavorable evolution of these patients. In addition, smoking can induce structural changes in the lungs, such as emphysema, which can lead to reduced lung function and greater vulnerability to respiratory infections (21). It therefore seems unlikely that this harmful substance would reduce the risk of contracting SARS-CoV-2 (11).

According to several studies, active or weaned smokers are at greater risk of developing severe forms of COVID-19 (11). According to a meta-analysis of 207 studies, smoking predicted mortality from COVID-19 with a high level of evidence (22). Zhao et al. analyzed data from 7 studies involving 1,726 patients and found a statistically significant association between smoking and the severity of COVID-19 (23). The same association was found by Zheng et al. who analyzed data from 5 studies with a total of 1980 patients (24). Vardavas et al. analyzed data from 5 studies totalling 1549 patients and found a correlation between smoking status and ICU admission, ventilation and death (25).

In contrast, a few studies found no significant association between smoking and the severity of SARS-CoV-2 infection, but these involved a small number of patients ranging from 11 to 145 (26). In our study, there was no correlation between smoking and the clinical severity of COVID-19 pneumonia, nor between the need for resuscitation and death.

This discrepancy in results in the literature is explained on the one hand by the multitude of classifications of the severity of SARS-CoV-2 respiratory involvement, with several proposed thresholds for SpO2 below which infection is considered severe, and by the existence of numerous prognostic factors for COVID-19 pneumopathy apart from smoking (22).

Radiologically, data in the literature have shown that CT lesions are similar in smokers and non-smokers, with ground-glass sometimes associated with predominantly peripheral and subpleural condensations (27). Some studies have shown that the extent of these lesions may be greater in non-smokers, such as a Turkish study involving 121 patients (28) and a Chinese study of 86 patients (29). This could be explained by the loss of pulmonary elasticity caused by smoking, which increases vulnerability to infection. Contrary to these data, other studies have found no link between smoking and the extent of radiological lesions (30). In our study, the extent of radiological lesions - ground-glass in 81.29% of cases and condensation in 54.8% - was similar in both groups.

CONCLUSIONS

CONCLUSION S

Although smoking is a known risk factor for respiratory disease and lung infection, the relationship between smoking and the severity of COVID-19 respiratory involvement remains ambiguous.

In this context, we carried out a retrospective descriptive study involving 237 patients who were hospitalized for COVID-19 pneumopathy in the Pneumology Department at Mohamed Taher Maamouri Nabeul Hospital during the period from September 2020 to March 2021. The aim of our study was to evaluate the impact of smoking on the radio clinical presentation of COVID-19 pneumopathy and to specify its influence on its evolution.

The study population was divided into two groups (G1 non-smoking group of 184 patients and G2 smoking group of 53 patients).

Our population was more male than female, with a sex ratio of 1.17. The smoking group was predominantly male, while the non-smoking group was predominantly female. The average age of our population was 62.7 ±13.7 years with no statically significant difference between the two groups (p=0.322). For the group of smokers, the average tobacco consumption was 33±22 PA [2 - 100 PA].

Obesity was present in 38.8% of cases, and more frequently in the first group (p=0.015). There was no statically significant difference between the two groups in the presence of diabetes (p=0.307), hypertension (p=0.11), heart failure (p=0.689), arrhythmia (p=0.323) and coronary insufficiency (0.317).

Fever and chest pain were more common among smokers, while the frequency of asthenia, dry cough, dyspnea, digestive signs, agueusia and anosmia was comparable between the two groups.

Roughly half of the cases (109 cases, 46%) were severe forms (defined as room air SpO2 below 90% and/or signs of respiratory struggle), with no significant difference between the two groups (p=0.845).

The main CT abnormalities found were ground glass (126 cases; 81.29%) and condensations (85 cases; 54.8%) of peripheral and subpleural distribution. The extent of lesions was comparable between smokers and non-smokers.

Both groups required oxygen therapy with an equivalent flow rate (G1 8.7±9.2 l/min versus G2 11.2 ±13.2 l/min; p=0.124) and Dexamethasone-based systemic corticosteroid therapy with a similar duration (G1 10.5±5.7 days versus G2 11.5 ±8.6 days; p=0.337).

Bronchial superinfection with recourse to antibiotic therapy was more frequent in the smoking group (G1 24 cases (13%), G2 15 cases (28.3%) ; p=0.008), while pulmonary embolism and cardiac complications were equally frequent between the two groups (G1 37 cases (20.1%) versus G2 5 cases (9.4%); p=0.073), (G1 21 cases (11.4%), G2 4 cases (7.5%); p=0.419).

Death rates and ICU stays were similar for both groups.

According to the data in our study, smoking status had no influence on the radio-clinical presentation of COVID-19 pneumopathy, nor on its evolutionary course. Nevertheless, smoking is the main risk factor for respiratory and cardiovascular comorbidities, which are important prognostic factors in this viral disease. Smoking cessation must therefore be one of the mainstays of treatment for all smokers who consult a health facility for SARS-CoV-2 infection, whatever its severity.

REFERENCES

REFERENCES

1 Garnier M, Quesnel C, Constantin JM. COVID-19-related lung disease. Presse Médicale Form. Feb 2021;2(1):14-24.

2. Muller M, Bulubas I, Vogel T. Prognostic factors in Covid-19. Npg. oct 2021;21(125):304-12.

3. Thomas D, Berlin I. Covid-19 and smoking. Arch Mal Coeur Vaiss Prat. Jan 2021;2021(294):26-9.

4. WHO-2019-nCoV-clinical-2021.2-fre.pdf. Available at: https://iris.who.int/bitstream/handle/10665/352279/WHO-2019-nCoV-clinical-2021.2-fre.pdf

5. Khalil A, Fartoukh M, Tassart M, Parrot A, Marsault C, and Carette MF. Role of MDCT in Identification of the Bleeding Site and the Vessels Causing Hemoptysis. AJR Am J Roentgenol. 2007 Feb;188(2):W117-25.

6. Lodé B, Jalaber C, Orcel T, Morcet-Delattre T, Crespin N, Voisin S, et al. Imaging of COVID-19 pneumonia. J Imag Diagn Interv. Sept 2020;3(4):249-58.

7. COVID-19 epidemiological update - 19 January 2024 . Available at: https://www.who.int/publications/m/item/covid-19-epidemiological-update---19-january-2024

8 WHO report on the global tobacco epidemic 2023. Disponible sur: https://iris.who.int/bitstream/handle/10665/372570/9789240077508-fre.pdf

9. Guan W jie, Ni Z yi, Hu Y, Liang W hua, Ou C quan, He J xing, et al. Clinical Characteristics of Coronavirus Disease 2019 in China. N Engl J Med. Apr 30, 2020;382(18):1708-20.

10. Miyara M, Tubach F, Pourcher V, Morelot-Panzini C, Pernet J, Haroche J, et al. Low incidence of daily active tobacco smoking in patients with symptomatic COVID-19. Apr 20, 2020; Available at: https://www.qeios.com/read/WPP19W.2

11. Simons D, Shahab L, Brown J, Perski O. The association of smoking status with SARS-CoV-2 infection, hospitalization and mortality from COVID-19: a living rapid evidence review with Bayesian meta-analyses (version 7). Addiction. 2021;116(6):1319-68.

12. Van Westen-Lagerweij NA, Meijer E, Meeuwsen EG, Chavannes NH, Willemsen MC, Croes EA. Are smokers protected against SARS-CoV-2 infection (COVID-19)? The origins of the myth. Npj Prim Care Respir Med. 26 Feb 2021;31(1):1-3.

13. Farsalinos K, Barbouni A, Niaura R. Systematic review of the prevalence of current smoking among hospitalized COVID-19 patients in China: could nicotine be a therapeutic option? Intern Emerg Med. August 2020;15(5):845-52.

14. Changeux JP, Amoura Z, Rey FA, Miyara M. A nicotinic hypothesis for Covid-19 with preventive and therapeutic implications. C R Biol. June 5, 2020;343(1):33-9.

15. Tizabi Y, Getachew B, Copeland RL, Aschner M. Nicotine and the nicotinic cholinergic system in COVID-19. FEBS J. 2020;287(17):3656-63.

16. Dratcu L, Boland X. Does Nicotine Prevent Cytokine Storms in COVID-19? Cureus. 12(10):e11220.

17. Farsalinos K, Niaura R, Le Houezec J, Barbouni A, Tsatsakis A, Kouretas D, et al. Editorial: Nicotine and SARS-CoV-2: COVID-19 may be a disease of the nicotinic cholinergic system. Toxicol Rep. 30 Apr 2020;7:658-63.

18. Oakes JM, Fuchs RM, Gardner JD, Lazartigues E, Yue X. Nicotine and the renin-angiotensin system. Am J Physiol-Regul Integr Comp Physiol. nov 2018;315(5):R895-906.

19. Yue X, Basting TM, Flanagan TW, Xu J, Lobell TD, Gilpin NW, et al. Nicotine Downregulates the Compensatory Angiotensin-Converting Enzyme 2/Angiotensin Type 2 Receptor of the Renin-Angiotensin System. Ann Am Thorac Soc. Apr 2018;15(Supplement_2):S126-7.

20. Cai G, Bossé Y, Xiao F, Kheradmand F, Amos CI. Tobacco Smoking Increases the Lung Gene Expression of ACE2, the Receptor of SARS-CoV-2. Am J Respir Crit Care Med. June 15, 2020;201(12):1557-9.

21. Rosoff DB, Yoo J, Lohoff FW. Smoking is significantly associated with increased risk of COVID-19 and other respiratory infections. Commun Biol. 28 Oct 2021;4:1230.

22. Izcovich A, Ragusa MA, Tortosa F, Marzio MAL, Agnoletti C, Bengolea A, et al. Prognostic factors for severity and mortality in patients infected with COVID-19: A systematic review. PLOS ONE. 17 Nov 2020;15(11):e0241955.

23. Zhao Q, Meng M, Kumar R, Wu Y, Huang J, Lian N, et al. The impact of COPD and smoking history on the severity of COVID-19: A systemic review and meta-analysis. J Med Virol.2020 Oct;92(10):1915-1921

24. Zheng Z, Peng F, Xu B, Zhao J, Liu H, Peng J, et al. Risk factors of critical & fatal COVID-19 cases: A systematic literature review and meta-analysis. J Infect. August 2020;81(2):e16-25.

25. Vardavas CI, Nikitara K. COVID-19 and smoking: A systematic review of the evidence. Tob Induc Dis. 2020;18:20.

26. WHO-2019-nCoV-Sci_Brief-Smoking-2020.2-eng.pdf. Available at: https://iris.who.int/bitstream/handle/10665/332895/WHO-2019-nCoV-Sci_Brief-Smoking-2020.2-eng.pdf?sequence=1

27. Chung M, Bernheim A, Mei X, Zhang N, Huang M, Zeng X, et al. CT Imaging Features of 2019 Novel Coronavirus (2019-nCoV). Radiology. 4 Feb 2020;200230.

28. Yağcı B, Özlem Balık A, Balık R, Yalım Uncu U. Can Thorax Computed Tomography Severity Score in Coronavirus Disease 2019 Patients Differentiate Smokers from Non-smokers? Turk Thorac J. March 1, 2022;23(2):130-7.

29. Xie X, Zhong Z, Zhao W, Wu S, Liu J. The Differences and Changes of Semi-Quantitative and Quantitative CT Features of Coronavirus Disease 2019 Pneumonia in Patients With or Without Smoking History. Frontiers in Medicine.Sep 8, 2021

30. Hasweh R, Khlaifat GS, Obeidat BN, Khabaz AA, Ghanayem MB, Al-Zioud LF, et al. Radiological Differences in COVID-19 Related Lung Manifestations Between Smokers and Non-smokers: A Single-Center Retrospective Study in Jordan. Cureus. 15(5):e38437.

APPENDIX

APPENDIX

Appendix 1: Worksheet

Matricule :....................DM : .... Entered on : ....../....../...... Released on: ....../......./...........
Number of hospital days: .... jrs
First and last name: .... **Gender:** M F

Date of birth:......................... ....Age: ....

Occupation: CM CS Worker Workplace: ....

Health profession: Yes No If Yes: Doctor Nurse Worker Administration

Telephone:........................... ....Email:...

Address:............................ ....

Active smoking Yes .... PA No Cannabis

Weaned : Yes since ...... No

Blood type :......................... ....

Vaccinated yes no

If yes: type of vaccine ....

- two doses with a delay of more than 3 weeks between the second injection and the date of confirmation of infection
- a single dose or less than 3 weeks between the second injection and the date of confirmation of infection

Interrogation :

❖ **History:**

▪ **Family :**

Diabetes Coronary heart diseaseHTA Asthma Atopy
Other:.................................. ....

▪ **Personnel :**

- Infection COVID 19 YES NO
- Respiratory: Yes No If YES: Asthma COPD DDB
- stage IRC pulmonary embolism OR DVT (delay since this episode = ...)
  Other:................................ ....

- Cardiovascular: Yes No If yes: hypertension heart failure
  Coronary insufficiency ACFA
- Diabetes: YES NO
- Insulino Necessary YES NO
- Renal insufficiency: YES NO
- Cirrhosis: YES NO
- Long-term treatment: YES NO
  Long-term corticosteroid therapy IS ACE inhibitors ARB II

  NSAIDs PAAs DTC anticoagulants hormonal contraception

- ***Gynaeco-obstetrics:***
  Pregnancy in progress: YES No

  Menopause Yes No

- BCG vaccination: YES No
- Drug allergy: YES No

❖ **Symptoms present :**

- No symptoms
- Duration of symptoms before consultation.........
- Headache Anorexia Asthenia/fatigue
- Weight loss Fever > 37.5° Chills
- Dry cough
- Arthralgia Myalgia
- Nausea and/or vomiting Abdominal pain
- Diarrhea
- Dyspnea Oppression and/or chest pain
- Odynophagia rash Rhinorrhea or nasal congestion
- Eye redness Confusion
- Agueusia Anosmia
- Other:...
- Diagnpstic confimré par PCR ; test rapide , Date .../......../.............
  <u>**Clinical examination:**</u> Weight: ....Height: ....IMC: ....

▪ Fever at start or during hospitalization (other than bacterial cpc) yes no

▪ **Neurological :**
Consciousness: Normal Confusion

▪ **Respiratory :**
FR :..........c/min

Signs of struggle: Yes No

Lung auscultation: Normal Abnormal RR RS RC

SpO2 (AA):........................

▪ **Cardiovascular :**
FC :........................

AC: normal Abnormal Breathing Irregular rhythm

Orthopnea: Yes No

IMO: Yes No

Spontaneous turgor (VJ): Yes No

Signs of phlebitis Yes No

- **Rash:** Yes No Describe: ....
- **Exmaen of gonglionary areas**
- **Abdominal examination**
  Normal sensitive specify location

  HMG SMG

- **Signs of dehydration** Yes No
  <u>**Additional tests :**</u>

- **GDS :** AA O_2 Flow rate :...

- pH = ...- PaO2 = ...mmHg - PaCO2 = ...mmHg - HCO3- = ...mmol/l -

  Sat O2 = ...% Lactate:..........

- **Biology on admission**

  NFS :GB :............PNN :................Lymph :...............HB :................

  VGM :.................. TCMH :................ .Plq :..

  CRP: ....

  Urea :.................... Créat :................. Cl Créat :.................................... ASAT :.................

  ALAT :............... □GT :..

  If cytolysis (ASAT...........N) ; (ALAT.............N)

  PAL :.................. .Bili T :.............. Conj :..

  Na+ :................... K+ :.................... Cl :..

  CPK :.................. LDH :................ D-dimer :.................................

  Troponins: 1er point :.....................2ème point :.........................3ème point :................

  DDIMERES initial ....

  If ascending during hospitalization, specify value ....

  If decrease during hospitalization, specify value ....

  Biology at discharge (if initial abnormality)

  CRP............. LYMPHOCYTE

  ASAT................ALAT...................

- **Initial chest x-ray: done not done**

  Normal Abnormal

  Unilobar Plurilobar

  Associated pleural: Yes No

  Syndrome: alveolar Interstitial Alveolo interstitial

- **Initial ECG:** QTc..........................ms
- **Initial chest CT:** not done Normal Abnormal

1) Extent of damage

   Absent minimal (< 10%) moderate (10-25%) extensive (25-50%)

   severe (50-75%) critical (>75%)

2) type of lesions

   frosted glass alone condensation alone frosted glass and condensation

   nodular lesions halot sign inverted halot sign

3) Lesion distribution

   Bilateral unilateral

   Subpleural peripheral predominance

Superior dominance

4) Associated radiological signs
mediastinal adenopathy

unilateral pleurisy bilateral pleurisy pneumothorax (treated by drainage yes no) pneumomediastinum

pericardial effusion

Pulmonary embolism: proximal distal

Unilateral bilateral

Complications

- □ Persistent dry cough if so, specify treatment□ cough syrup (specify...........);□ ICS
- □ Bacterial superinfection
  Type of antibiotic therapy received ....
  Duration of antibiotic therapy....................
  ECBC made no made
  If cultured: positive negative
  If positive: germ type ....
- □ Inflammatory anemia (hb<13 male; <12 female) with elevated ferritinemia
- □ Thrombocytosis(> 450,000/mcL)
- □ Functional renal failure

- □ Cardiac complications
  - o Rhythm disorder if yes, specify ....
  - o Acute coronary syndrome
  - o IC surge
  - o Pericardial effusion

- □ Hyponatremia (Na<135 confirmed by two samples)
  Lowest Na figures...............;
  urinary iono Nau< 20 / Nau>20
- • Treatment: water restriction
- • Salt intake
- □ Hyperkalemia> 5.5 confirmed by iono without tourniquet outside of acute CKD
- □ Pulmonary embolism: proximal distal
  Unilateral bilateral

- □ Deep vein thrombosis
  If PE or DVT
  - o Occurrence on preventive anticoagulant therapy
  - o Occurrence on curative anticoagulant therapy
- □ Arterial complication; specify ....

- □ Bleeding (specify.................) , following curative anticoagulant therapy□ yes □no
- □ Tares imbalance
  - o Diabetes imbalance
    - ▪ With acidosis
    - ▪ No acidosis
  - o Exacerbation of chronic respiratory diseases
  - o HTA imbalance
  - o Decompensation of psychiatric pathology

- Others............................
- Discovering little-known defects
- HTA
- Diabetes
- Other................
- Nosocomial complications
  Eschar
  Infection
- Confusion

Treatment

1) Initial O2 flow............l/mn (<6l/mn >6l/mn)
2) Corticosteroid therapy
   Prescribed molecule...
   Initial dose ....
   Secondary increase .... ; cause...............dose ....
   Total duration CT...
3) Anticoagulation
- Preventive
- Curative
  If curative anticoagulation, specify indication

- Thromboembolic complication
- Heart rhythm disorder or ACS without thromboembolic complications

4) Azithromycin yes no
- Received prior to hospitalization
- Received during hospitalization
  duration ....

5) Vitamin D yes no
6) Vitamin C yes no
7) Zinc yes no

Evolution

- Number of days of oxygen therapy ....
- Number of hospital days ....
- SpO2 at output ....AA
- Exit without oxygen
- Output with oxygen
- Transfer to intensive care
- Deaths
- Discharge on preventive anticoagulation O AOD O LMWH
  Total duration of preventive anticoagulation .... (excluding long-term curative indications)

Selected diagnosis

- Paucisymptomatic SARS COV 2 infection
- Minor SARS VOC infection
- Moderate SARS COV 2 infection
- Moderate to severe SARS COV 2 infection
- Severe SARS COV2 infection

Impact of smoking on the radioclinical presentation and evolution of COVID-19 pneumonitis

Summary

Introduction: The 2019 coronavirus pandemic (COVID-19) caused by *Severe Acute Respiratory Syndrome-Coronavirus 2* was responsible for high morbidity and mortality. Several prognostic factors have been identified, but the impact of smoking on this condition remains controversial.

Methods: Retrospective descriptive study involving patients who were hospitalized for COVID-19 pneumopathy in the Pneumology Department at Mohamed Taher Maamouri Hospital, Nabeul, from September 2020 to March 2021. The main objective of our study was to evaluate the impact of smoking on the radio clinical presentation of this condition and its evolutionary course.

Results: Our population consisted of 237 patients with a mean age of 62.7 years and a sex ratio of 1.17. The study population was divided into two groups: G1, a group of non-smoking patients (184 patients), and G2, a group of smoking patients (53 patients). G1 was predominantly female, while G2 was predominantly male. The two groups were comparable in terms of age, presence of diabetes, hypertension, heart failure, arrhythmia and coronary insufficiency, but obesity was more frequent in the first group (p=0.015). Fever and chest pain were more frequent in smokers, while the frequency of asthenia, dry cough, dyspnea and digestive signs was similar for G1 and G2. The percentage of severe forms was similar for smokers and non-smokers. There was no statistically significant difference in the extent of ground-glass and condensation lesions on CT, nor in the oxygen flow rate required, nor in the duration of corticosteroid therapy prescribed. Rates of death and ICU stay were similar for both groups.

Conclusion: Smoking does not appear to have any impact on the radio-clinical presentation of COVID-19 pneumopathy, nor on its evolutionary course. Nevertheless, tobacco control should be a major concern for all clinicians, given its undoubted role in respiratory and cardiovascular co-morbidities, which are poor prognostic factors in all infectious lung diseases.

Key words: COVID-19, Smoking, Prognosis

Impact of smoking on the radio-clinical presentation and evolution of COVID-19 pneumonia

Abstract

Introduction:

The coronavirus disease 2019 (COVID-19) pandemic caused by *Severe Acute Respiratory Syndrome-Coronavirus 2* was responsible for high morbidity and mortality. Several prognostic factors have been identified, but the impact of smoking on this disease remains controversial.

Methods:

Retrospective descriptive study of patients hospitalized with COVID-19 pneumonia in the Pneumology Department at Mohamed Taher Maamouri Hospital, Nabeul, from September 2020 to March 2021. The main objective of our study was to evaluate the influence of smoking on the radio-clinical presentation of this disease and its evolutionary course.

Results:

Our population consisted of 237 patients with a mean age of 62.7 years and a sex ratio of 1.17. The study population was divided into two groups: G1, a group of non-smoking patients (184 patients), and G2, a group of smoking patients (53 patients). G1 was predominantly female, while G2 was predominantly male. The two groups were comparable in terms of age, presence of diabetes, arterial hypertension, heart failure, arrhythmia and coronary insufficiency, but obesity was more frequent in the first group ($p=0.015$). Fever and chest pain were more common in smokers, while asthenia, dry cough, dyspnoea and digestive signs were similar in G1 and G2. The percentage of severe forms was similar for smokers and non-smokers. There were no statistically significant differences in the extent of ground-glass and condensation lesions on scans, the oxygen flow rate required or the duration of corticosteroid therapy. The rates of death, intensive care unit stay and discharge on oxygen were similar for the two groups.

Conclusion:

Smoking does not appear to have any impact on the radio-clinical presentation of COVID-19 pneumonia, or on its course. Nevertheless, the fight against smoking should be a major concern for all clinicians, given its undoubted role in respiratory and cardiovascular co-morbidities, which are factors in the poor prognosis of any infectious pneumopathy.

Keywords: COVID-19, Smoking, Prognosis

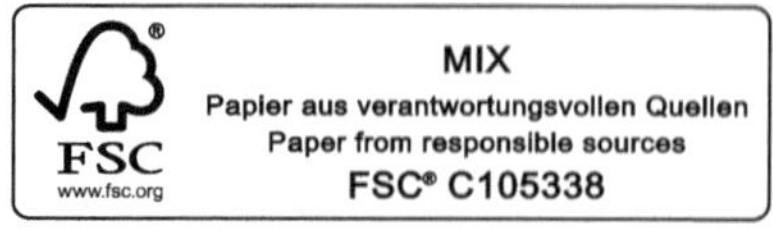

Printed by Books on Demand GmbH, Norderstedt / Germany